Herbal Antibiotics:

25 Homemade Remedies for Healing

Table of Contents

In a world of prescription drugs, you're looking for something else…

Yes, pharmacopeia as advanced, but with every medication from the laboratory that's been tested and released to the public, there are side-effects that can make you cringe and apprehensive about even taking the medicine. You're wondering if there are any other ways to maintain your health and also how to treat illnesses like colds, flu and other viruses and infections. There is. In the holistic world, there are herbs and essential oils, as well as grains and foods that can prevent illness or treat them if you happen to bring one home from work.

There is a lot of information on the internet and books, and your head is spinning from all the advice and recipes you have found. You have no idea what half of those are supposed to do, let alone what to expect when taking them. This book puts it in an easy format to follow.

Chapter 1 – Your immune system and holistic health.

Holistic health does not focus on the symptoms of illnesses. Rather, it focuses on the root cause and treats it from a whole-body and mind perspective. This means, holistic medicine takes into account that everyone's body is different and metabolizes food, medicine and other substances ingest differently as well. While some of you may need a full dose, others may only need a half-dose.

Holistic medicine also takes into consideration what you are eating and how your' body handles outside influences, such as stress and the environment around you. All these factor into the illness you have and how to go about treating it properly. Dietary changes, coping with outside influences, and talking remedies are all included in holistic healing practices.

It's starts with your Immune system

Your immune system is the front-line soldier to all the viruses and infections the environment throws at you. It springs into action when the smallest of invaders tries to take over. There are factors to take into consideration which can contribute to your immune system being weakened.

Sleep

Your body needs six to eight hours of quality sleep. Quality sleep means waking up in the morning rested and full of energy to face the day. Breaking the sleep cycle, insomnia, and constantly tossing and turning reduces your quality of sleep, and can weaken the immune system.

When you rest your head for the night, make sure you haven't ingested any caffeinated products, as these drinks can prevent your body from relaxing completely, allowing you to fall asleep. Also make sure you can dedicate at least six hours of sleep to get the minimum amount of rest.

Diet

In this world where everything needs to be done yesterday means your grabbing the quickest eats and snacks on your way to, or from, work and home. Foods that are highly processed and laden with artificial additives compromise your nutrition, and can contribute to having your immune system not working as it should.

This can be reduced by reading ingredients and avoiding anything laden with artificial colors, flavors, and preservatives. The closer you get to the way the food is supposed to be, the longer you will feel full, and your body will get the nutrients your body will need to feed your immune system.

Plan your meals and snacks ahead and package them in containers for easy travel and quick heating. It may take a little getting used to at first, but your body will thank you in the long run.

Stress

Bill paying, running around to do chores, and your daily work load can all cause stress. If your married, trying to raise children and keeping up with their schedules can also add to your stress levels. Constantly being in stressful situations can put kinks in your immune system , causing you to be more prone to getting sick.

There are many ways to cope with stress, increase your endorphins, and reduce your chances of contracting an illness.

1. Take time out for yourself. Just one-half hour to one hour just for doing what you want to do. This can be reading a book, writing in a journal, or even taking a long bath. Taking time out for you makes you feel better and

relaxes your body and mind, letting your immune system regain some of its strength.

2. Try deep breathing. Deep breathing and meditation helps you to shake off the day's trials and stresses. This, in turn, helps your mind relax and your body as well. Meditation and deep breathing has been proven to reduce stress and anxiety.

3. Exercise. This leads into the next point. So, I won't go much into it in this list.

4. Unplug. Between the television, the computer, and your smart phone, you are constantly bombarding your mind with stimulus it's trying to cope with and dissimilate. Instead of answering that text or replying to that email or Facebook post, unplug and turn off the electronics and allow your mind to come down from all information you're constantly feeding it. Relaxing your brain relaxes your body.

Stagnant lifestyle

A lifestyle where you don't get the minimum amount of physical activity can also contribute to a weaker immune system. Exercise helps to boost the action of the lymph nodes in the immune system, making it easier for them to cleanse themselves. When you lead a stagnant lifestyle, your lymph nodes accumulate toxins they can't get rid of, thus making it more likely that you will get sick.

I am not telling you to start going to a gym and sweating until you can't move. Exercise can be as easily as going for a walk in a park or down your street. Yoga, Qi Gong, and Tai Chi all are all good forms of low-impact activities that can help you lower your stress, get those endorphins flowing and boost your immune system.

Just twenty minutes a day can get you on your way to a healthier you.

Chapter 2 – Herbal antibiotics and immune boosters

For every illness, there is an herb to help the body get rid of it. Your body is an amazing self-healing machine, but even it needs help from time to time. There are herbal supplements, teas, and other remedies than can help boost the immune system to help you prevent illness and herbal antibiotics for when you find yourself in the middle of fighting an infection or virus.

The two lists below are broken into antibiotics and immune system boosters. Though they can work beautifully together, if you don't need to take antibiotics when you are not fighting an infection or virus you can leave to the side, but first, we will explain the difference between infections and viruses.

There are viral infections and bacterial infections

Viral infections, such as the flu and the common cold, cannot be treated with antibiotics. Bacterial infections can be treated by antibiotics. You can run fevers with both, and that is perfectly normal. A fever is your body's way of burning out a virus or infection. This means taking anything to reduce the fever can reduce your body's ability to fight the illness. If your fever goes past 102, I would highly recommend going to a physician, but anything under that can be burned out or broken by sweating it out.

Sweating out a fever

Take a hot shower and get dressed in warm clothing and cover yourself up to your head. Stay under the covers until you break the fever. This usually a few hours to do, and your sheets will be drenched in sweat, but the fever will be broken and you can now go about being more aggressive in treating your illness.

What is aggressively treating an illness?

This is the act of outwardly and internally treating an illness. To break it down further, it's the practice of ingesting remedies while using topical remedies at the same time. This is a dual-fronted way of attacking an illness. It is effective in shortening the time you are ill and speeds up healing time.

Herbal Antibiotics

Herbal antibiotics, unlike the one you get from the doctor, attack the bacterial infection causing the illness, and not everything they consider an infection. Most, if not all, prescription antibiotics attack anything it considers bacteria. This includes the probiotics that help with digestion and boost the immune system.

-Acacia (acacia arabica)

This herb is usually sold in powder form. However, the bark can be boiled and used to gargle for infections of the mouth, and to help treat most types of food poisoning, which stems from bacterial infections.

-Aloe (aloe vera)

Though more often used to treat burns and cuts, when aloe is taken in small doses as a drink, it can help to treat bacterial infections. It also helps to increase the appetite in those who have lost it due to illness or some medications.

-Echinacea (echinacea purpurea)

More commonly thought of as an immune system booster, Echinacea also has antibacterial and antiviral properties as well. It can be taken as a tea, capsule, tincture, or extract. Some have even included it in herbal baths with other antivirals.

Eucalyptus (eucalyptus globulus)

When you hear the name of this herb, many think of respiratory herbs. You aren't wrong, but it is also antibacterial. it also helps the body to expel phlegm.

Garlic (allium sativum)

This is one of the kings of the herbal and cooking world. It is also an adaptogen, meaning it assess the body's needs and shore up weaknesses. It is also a strong antibacterial.

Ginger (zingiber officinale)

This is a catalyst and binding herb with antibacterial properties. This means it actually helps to boost the actions of other herbs in the mix. It also helps to tie in all the herbs together in the combination.

Goldenseal (hydrastis canadensis)

Also known as Yellow Root, this herb has been used for killing bacteria and treating infections and infected wounds. You can include it in syrups and decoctions. Proceed with caution if you have low blood sugar, though. It has a tendency to make blood sugar levels drop.

Juniper Berries (juniperus species)

Yes, you can find this herb in the US in a lot of yards as ground cover, but the berries can be juiced or made into a tea to fight bacterial infections. It has also been known to regulate blood sugar levels; so, beware if you are taking insulin or are a diabetic.

Licorice Root (glycyrrhiza glabra)

Yes, this is the same licorice in natural licorice candies. It has been known to also fight infections and helps the body get rid of bacteria. Don't take it in large doses, because it can cause diarrhea.

These herbs, as the title of the section states, helps to shore up, fortify, and boost the action of the immune system. When you boost the immune system, you decrease the severity and duration of infections and viruses.

Cat's Claw (unicaria tomentosa)

This rain forest herb is five times more effective than Echinacea in terms of immune system boosters. It is also a strong antiviral and can be used in teas, herbal baths, syrups, and cleansing baths.

Echinacea

I listed this above, but it can be used in teas, syrups, oils, and extracts.

Garlic

This herb is also a great immune booster. It has to be taken in small doses at first though. It does have a strong taste as well as smell and can induce vomiting, if your body is not used to eating it by itself.

Goldenseal

Also, from above, this herb is also known to boost the immune system and is also coupled with Echinacea in extracts and other products.

Antivirals

The flu and the common cold are viruses. They are infectious, but are not bacterial infections. Below are some herbs you can use to help fight these viruses.

-Calendula Petals (calendula officinalis)

Also known as Marigold, the petals of this annual flower have been used to help the body fight viruses and treat wounds.

-Echinacea

This herb is also a strong antiviral.

-Garlic

This is another property of this herb.

-Ginger

This is herb can be taken on its own and is also known to be added to home remedies to kick colds and viruses.

-Juniper Berries

This was mentioned above, but Juniper Berries also used in preparations to help the body fight viruses, too.

Chapter 3 – Essential oils

When you choose to aggressively fight a virus or bacterial infection, you need to also attack it from the topical sense as well. This means as massage oils, mineral baths, ointments, chest rubs, and a host of other preparations. Presenting a dual front to fight illness means you recognize you need to clean out the lymph nodes by either using a massage oil, mineral bath, or salve.

-Basil, French (ocimum basilicum)

This essential oil has been used to help the immune system. It is also a potent antiviral and can help to treat colds, flu, helps to break fevers, and also helps to stem coughs.

-Bergamot (citrus bergamia)

This essential helps fight internal and external infections, infections of the mouth, and also is used to strength the immune system to help the body fight colds and flu. It can also help in cases of communicable infectious diseases.

-Eucalyptus Blue Gum (eucalyptus globulus)

The essential oil of this herb can help to open respiratory passages. It's antiviral and antibiotic properties help to fight Chickenpox, colds, flu, measles and other viruses.

-Lavender (Lavandula angustifolia)

This essential oil is famous for its ability to treat burns, but it also has antiviral, antibacterial, and it can also boost the immune system. It can help with throat infections and the flu.

-Peppermint (mentha piperita)

This famous herb has an essential oil which is used to fight colds, flu, and to aid in breaking fevers. It has antiseptic and antiviral properties.

-Sage, Clary (salvia sclarea)

As an essential oil, it can used in external preparations to help treat throat infections, cleanse lymph nodes. and can help the body fight bacteria.

-Tea Tree (melaleuca alternifolia)

This immune system boosting essential oil is especially potent in killing bacteria, infections, and other illnesses like Chickenpox.

-Thyme, Common (thymus vulgaris)

This is another essential oil which is used for diseases like Chickenpox and measles. It can help to treat colds, flu, and other viruses and infections.

Word to the wise.

Essential oils should not be used without diluting them first. Undiluted essential oils can cause contact dermatitis. You will also need to go to a store which sells essential oils to perform a patch test to make sure you are not sensitive to the essential oils before using them.

Base/carrier oils

The most common carrier oils, oils you dilute essentials into, are Sweet Almond Oil or Apricot Kernel Oil. You can use vegetable oil if you do not want to go out and buy a carrier oil. You can also use olive oil, but you would need to mix it with another oil.

Chapter 4 – Foods that help with illness

There are foods you can eat during recovering from an illness that can give your body a fighting chance. Conversely, there are foods you would need to stay away from to better your chances to bounce back from an illness.

Foods to avoid

When you have an illness that produces mucous, staying away from dairy or whole wheat foods can help speed up recovery time. These two foods produce mucous in the body, which can make respiratory viruses worse or lengthen the illness time.

Highly processed foods are often not the foods you need to ingest while you are trying to kick a virus or bacterial infection. These types of foods often are not nutrient-rich foods that can further boost your immune system.

Foods to help heal

When you are ill, the hardest thing to do is eat. You are not very hungry, but you need to eat to feed your immune system the fuel it needs to fight the illness.

Super Foods

These are foods that are nutrient rich can be added to other foods to help speed recovery. Some of these foods are the following:

-Spirulina

This super food can be taken by capsules. It is rich in vitamins and minerals and has natural detoxing properties that can help the body kick a virus or infections.

-Colored foods

Carrots, bell peppers, blueberries, strawberries and foods that are brightly colored have antioxidants to help your body fight illnesses.

-Kombucha tea

This can be purchased as a starter kit. This mushroom has strong antiviral and immune system boosting properties.

Kefir, both water and dairy grain

Kefir grains are cultures that contain more than 200 probiotics than all the yogurt on the market put together. You can purchase the grains online and they come with instructions. Kefir, by replenishing the friendly bacteria in your system, can boost your immune system and help to speed recovery from viruses and bacterial infections.

Chapter 5 – Recipes to help speed healing

We all have recipes we love to make when we are sick. Comfort food is always reached for to make us feel better. Here are some recipes you may add to your menu the next time you're feeling under the weather.

Sick day juice

This juice may be a little potent in taste, but it gets the job done.

3 Cloves of garlic, pressed.

2 Tbsp of ginger, pressed.

1/2 Tsp Cayenne Pepper

1 medium organic tomato

1. Run the tomato through a juicer.

2. Add the first three ingredients.

3. Shake well and take like you would a shot of whiskey.

4. You can follow it up with a glass of orange juice to get the taste out of your mouth.

Antioxidant Juice

2 Medium Carrots

1 Small tomato

3 Celery Stalks

1/4 Cup Blueberries

1/4 Cup Strawberries

1 Medium Green Apple

1 Medium Orange

-Run all the ingredients through a juicer and drink in 4-ounce servings throughout the day.

Chicken Soup

Nothing beats a good chicken soup. We often turn to this comfort food when are feeling ill.

2 Boneless Skinless Chicken Breast. whole

3 Cloves of Garlic, minced

3 Tablespoons White Onion, minced

2 Tablespoons Rubbed Sage

1 Tablespoon Rosemary

1 Tablespoon Sea Salt

1 Medium Tomato, chopped

3 Medium Carrots, chopped

3 Stalks of Celery, chopped

1 Medium Sweet Potato, chopped

2 tsp Olive oil

Water

• Place the Olive Oil in the pot and gently heat it.

• Sauté the onion on medium heat and add the salt

• Add the Garlic and sauté.

• Add the cooking herbs and three tablespoons of water.

• Let it simmer for 5 minutes

• You can use either cornstarch, or flour here just to thicken.

• Add 32 Ounces of water, bring to a boil.

• Add the Chicken whole.

• Add the vegetables

• Periodically taste and add the herbs and salt to taste.

• When the chicken is cooked, take it out and chop it. Return it to the pot.

• You can, at this point, take the sweet potato and carrots and place them into a blender with a little bit of the stalk. Liquefy it and add it back to the soup. This will also help to thicken it.

Chapter 6 – Mineral Baths

Herbal and minerals baths can help speed healing. Many nutrients and medicinal properties of the herbs can be absorbed through the skin. Here are a few recipes you can use to help speed healing.

I will start out by listing the base recipes and then go on to listing what you can add the base to get the effect you are looking for. Once you add the other ingredients, add to running water in 1/4 cup increments.

Basic Mineral Bath Recipe I

1 Cup Sea Salt

1/2 Cup Epsom Salt

1/4 Cup Borax (This is a naturally occurring mineral and is packed with nutrients.)

1/4 Cup Baking Soda

• Mix all of these together and set aside.

Basic Mineral Bath Recipe II (For those who are hypertensive)

1 Cup of Ground Steel Cut Oats

1/2 Cup Borax

1/4 Cup Baking Soda

• Mix together and set aside

Basic Salts bath

2 Cups Sea Salt

1/2 ounce your choice of herbs.

• Mix together and set aside.

• Place 1/4 cup of the mixture in a reusable filter bag, preferably a quart size bag.

• Place the bag in a warm or hot bath and let the herbs make a tea in the water.

• To give your bath more punch, you can use the bag as a wash cloth to absorb more of the medicinal properties of the herbs.

Cold Bath

1/4 Cup Aloe Juice

10 Drops of Lavender essential oil

10 Drops of Eucalyptus essential oil

3 Drops of Sage essential oil

2 Drops of Thyme essential oil

• Mix all of the ingredients together.

• Can be used with the first two base recipes

• Once they are mix make sure you add them to the dry ingredients and place them in a tightly lidded container overnight to get the best effect.

Flu Bath

1/4 Cup Sweet Almond or Apricot Kernel oil

10 Drops of Peppermint essential oil

10 Drops of Bergamot essential oil

5 Drops of Tea Tree essential oil

• Mix all of them together and then follow the above directions.

• Can be used with the first two base recipes.

Antibiotic Bath

2 Ounces of Echinacea

2 Ounces of Juniper Berries

2 Ounces of Licorice Root

2 Ounces of Calendula petals

1/4 Cup of Sweet Almond oil

15 Drops of Eucalyptus essential oil

10 Drops of Lavender essential oil

5 Drops of French Basil

• Mix all of the dry ingredients and set aside

• Mix all of the oils together and set aside.

• Mix the herbs with base recipe number three

• Add the essential oil blend to the dry mixture

• Place the mixture in a tightly lidded container overnight.

• Use as the instructions for base recipe number three.

Antiviral Herbal Bath

This is different from the above recipes.

2 Ounces of Echinacea

2 Ounces of Calendula Petals

2 Ounces of Ginger root

2 Ounces of Cat's Claw

• Mix all of the herbs together.

• Boil the herbs in a large pot on the stove.

• Strain the plant material out.

• Add the tea to a bath full of water.

Chapter 7 -Infusions and Decoctions

In the world of herbal teas, there are two kinds: infusions and decoctions.

• Infusions are tea preparations that use petals and leaves of the plant. They are generally made by pour a quart of hot water through a strainer where an ounce of plant material is placed. You can also use normal measurements and machines (coffee or tea pot) to make infusions.

• Decoctions are tea preparations that use the roots, stems and seeds. These are boiled for fifteen minutes to extract the medicinal properties of the herbs used.

You can mix the two in order to make the herbs, but you would have to use a pot to do it. The best pots to use are porcelain or glass to prevent any contamination of the tea.

There are also two strengths: maintenance and therapeutic. The following recipes are therapeutic strength. To make them maintenance (everyday) strength, use one teaspoon of herbs per 6 ounces of water.

Antiviral Tea

1 Tbsp Echinacea

2 Tbsp Calendula

1 Tbsp Peppermint

1 Tbsp Licorice Root

• Simmer the Licorice Root for 15 minutes in 8 ounces of water.

• Place the rest of the ingredients in a coffee or tea filter

• Make a pot of tea.

• Add the Licorice to the pot

• Sweeten with organic raw honey

• You can also add lemon juice, if you desire.

Antibiotic Tea

1 Tbsp Ginger

1 Tbsp Juniper Berries

1 Tbsp Cat's Claw

1 Tbsp Eucalyptus

• Place all the herbs in a filter

• Boil the berries for 15 minutes

• Make a pot and add the berry decoction

Respiratory infection Tea

I am going to introduce a couple of new herbs here.

1 Tbsp Slippery Elm (Helps to bring up mucous from the lungs)

1 Tbsp Echinacea

1 Tbsp Mullein (Nutritionally strengthens the lungs.)

1 Tbsp Licorice Root Powder

1 Tbsp Catnip (Cough suppressant)

• Make a pot with the above ingredients.

Even though the goal for a respiratory infection is to get the infection out by coughing, adding the Catnip will prevent you from coughing constantly. The goal is to expel mucous without inflaming the chest wall, which causes pains in the chest when you breathe.

Sinusitis Tea

1 Tbsp Fenugreek seeds (Helps to break up impacted sinuses.)

1 Tbsp Thyme (Helps to fight the infection.)

1 Tbsp Echinacea

1 Tbsp Juniper Berries

1 Tbsp Mullein

• Boil the seeds and berries for 15 minutes in 8 ounces of water

• Make the rest of the tea as a half pot.

• Add the boiled seeds and berries to the pot.

Flu Tea

1 Tbsp Boneset powder (Breaks fevers)

1 Tbsp Echinacea

1 Tbsp Juniper Berries

2 Tbsp powdered Ginger

• Boil the Berries in 8 ounces of water for 15 minutes

• Make the pot of tea with the rest of the ingredients and add the berry decoction.

Chapter 8 - Salves, Oils, and Blends

In order to actively treat a virus or infection you also have to attack it from the outside. This means making salves, oils, essential oil blends.

Chest Salve

2 Tbsp Eucalyptus leaves

2 Tbsp Echinacea

1 Tbsp Juniper Berries

1 Tsp Peppermint Leaves

1 Tsp Ginger Root

2 Cups Olive or Apricot Kernel oil

1/4 Cup Beeswax beads

• Place the herbs and the oil in a crock pot on low overnight.

• Strain out the herbs

• In a Double boiler, melt the beeswax

• Add the infused oil

• Place in dark glass jars with tight lids.

• To use, rub an even amount on your chest and place plastic wrap on it so the medicine will be more readily absorbed.

Sinus salve

2 Tbsp Thyme

2 Tbsp Fenugreek seeds

1 Tbsp Eucalyptus Leaves

1 Tsp Ginger

1 Tsp Echinacea

1 Tsp Licorice Root

2 Cups Olive or Apricot Kernel oil

1/4 Cup Beeswax beads

• Follow the directions for the chest salve

• Apply to the sinus areas.

Antiviral Lymph Node oil

2 Tbsp Juniper Berries

2 Tbsp Echinacea

2 Tbsp Calendula Petals

4 Ounces of Olive or Apricot kernel oil

20 Drops Lavender essential oil

10 Drops Peppermint essential oil

5 Drops Thyme essential oil

5 Drops Sage essential oil

5 Drops Basil essential oil

5 Drops Eucalyptus essential oil

• Place the herbs and oil in a crock pot on low overnight.

• Strain the herbs out.

• Place in a dark glass or plastic bottle with a tight lid.

• When it cools, add the essential oil and mix well.

• Rub the oil into lymph nodes under your chin or any other place where your lymph nodes are swollen.

Diffuser Blends

These are blends you pre-mix and can place in either an essential oil diffuser or a candle warmer.

Immune Booster Blend

5 Drops Lavender essential oil

3 Drops Thyme

2 Drops Sage essential oil

Antiviral Blend

5 Drops Eucalyptus essential oil

3 Drops Tea Tree oil essential oil

2 Drops Bergamot essential oil

Cold and Flu Blend

5 Drops Lavender essential oil

3 Drops Peppermint essential oil

2 Drops Thyme essential oil

Antibacterial Spray

In order to prevent the spread of the virus, you need to kill it by sanitizing areas in your home where everyone comes in contact with it.

1 ounce cheap clear vodka

3 ounces distilled water

20 Drops Peppermint essential oil

20 Drops Tea Tree essential oil

10 Drops Bergamot essential oil

• Mix the essential oils with the vodka. This will help to mix the essential oils more effectively.

• Add the water.

• Pour into a spray bottle.

• Shake well and spray on surfaces.

• You can also use it as a cleanser and wipe it on the surfaces.

Chapter 9 Syrups

There will be times when you need a stronger herbal mix than tea. Here are a few herbal cough syrups.

To make the syrups:

• Place the herbs in a stock pot.

• Add a quart of water

• Boil down to a quart.

• Strain out the plant material

• Pour into a glass jar

• Add two ounces of honey or glycerin.

• Take a tablespoon every four hours.

Respiratory Syrup

1/2 Ounce of Slippery Elm

1/2 Ounce of Catnip

1/2 Ounce of Mullein

1/2 Ounce of Licorice or Wild Cherry Bark (Both are expectorants and both taste different)

Sinus Syrup

1/2 Ounce Fenugreek seeds

1/2 Ounce Thyme

1/2 Ounce Calendula petals

1/2 Ounce Echinacea

Cold and Flu Syrup

1/2 Ounce Calendula Petals

1/2 Ounce of Juniper Berries

1/2 Ounce of Peppermint

1/2 Ounce of Ginger

Conclusion

I hope this book has helped you, and spark a curiosity in your to make your own recipes. You can go online to find about more recipes, how to combine essential oils and herbals. There are communities online that are helpful and will answer any questions you have about natural health, herbalism, and aromatherapy.

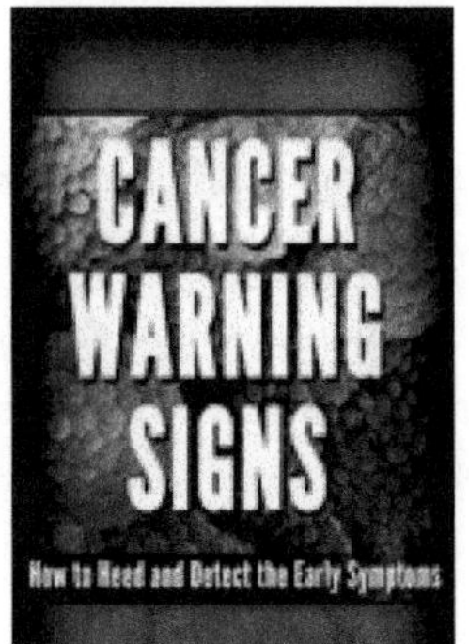

If you have not grabbed it yet, please go ahead and download your special bonus report *"Cancer Warning Signs. How To Heed & Detect The Early Symptoms!"*

Simply Click the Button Below

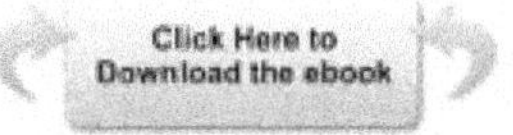

OR **Go to This Page**

http://healthylivingpeople.com/free/

BONUS #2: More Free & Discounted Books or Products

Do you want to receive more Free/Discounted Books or Products?

We have a mailing list where we send out our new Books or Products when they go free or with a discount on Amazon. Click on the link below to sign up for Free & Discount Book & Product Promotions.

=> Sign Up for Free & Discount Book & Product Promotions <=

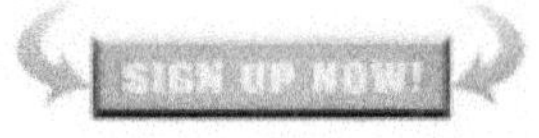

OR Go to this URL